<u>Societal Customs VS The Creators Diet Design</u>

Written By: Jessica Linhart

She firmly believes that we are one in Christ.

All Christians are a component of a community

where old socials standards of hierarchies and

gender divisions have no place in ministry.

(Joel 2:28; Acts 2:17 and 2 Cor. 5:17; Gal. 3:28)

Introduction: Why does my diet not work?

I believe that the Holy Spirit has given me the answer to this question. We worship God; which is a Trinity. God is the head, Jesus is the son, and the Holy Spirit is the comforter. Just like the Trinity of god, we are a three-part being. For example, we are first and foremost a spirit, we have a soul, but we live in a body. In addition, To live in this world we must have a body, because absent from the body is present with the Lord. As God's children, we must be fit in the spirit, soul, and body. Finally, a good diet does not work, because it has nothing to do with the spirit. Therefore, since we are a spiritual being with three parts, a weight loss plan, has to be a plan that includes the spirit, soul, and body.

Paul says in Scripture that he must bring his body into subjection. Just like Paul we can also bring our bodies into subjection, because we allow the spirit to God and direct paths. When we put the spirit first and it is saturated in nutrients; then, we can concentrate on the body. PraiseMoves works, because as we are working out; will you be building a relationship with God through the spirit. When our spirit is under subjection to God miraculous things occur. Moreover, scripture says for us to come out of the world. We do not need to look like the world. We should be different! Our demeanors and attributes should be different and we should set an example for all those to see God.

In addition, For me, comfort came from food. I

enjoyed eating above everything else. When I quit

eating like the world I obtained my comfort from

God and lost weight.

Chapter 1: What did God give us to eat?

Today's text comes from **Genesis 1:29-30** " And God said, Behold, I have given you every herb bearing seed, which is upon the face of all the earth, and every tree, in the which is the fruit of a tree yielding seed; to you it shall be for meat. 30And to every beast of the earth, and to every fowl of the air, and to every thing that creepeth upon the earth, wherein there is life, I have given every green herb for meat: and it was so.

God made it very simple, because he wanted us to live healthy lives. Creator God gave all plant life that yields a seed to us and the animals for food. Mankind decided that other things tasted good; therefore, we began to eat differently. Thus, mankind created it's own custom for societal

eating.

Chapter 2: What is God's diet plan for me?

To begin explaining the answer to the Gist chapters question we can first begin by opening the Bible to book one. Book one is Genesis. In the first chapter we read that God created everything and had a specific set of instructions he followed. God created mankind in his image and he designed us so that we would have to consume a certain amount of calories each day. I was really really down this pages of genesis we find that God created all plant life and vegetation. Yes, we as mankind, are supposed to eat and be partakers of plant life and the vegetation of the world.

You know, when I first began looking at my unhealthy lifestyle, I questioned how did I end up this way. I am a true believer, I thought. Therefore,

if I'm a true believer; then, why I'm I not studying

Scripture and learning God's diet plan?

I realized that I was holding the best diet plan

in the world; which, is the Bible. As believers, God

called us out of the world to live separately from

the world (**2 Corinthians 6:17**). I thought I was

doing that, but I hadn't inspected my diet. I was

eating mostly fast food, packaged items, and

drinking a lot of soda. Then, as I began to study

essential oils and the vegetation of the world I

realized that I was considering God's products. For

example, I enjoy eating raw carrots, but when I cut

a carrot in half I recognized that I had two eyes

gazing back at me. Then, as I began examining the appearance of other veggies; such as, celery, I comprehended that it's shape resembled the shape of my bones. Finally, I'm sharing this with you, because God made all of His produce in the shape of the things that we are familiar with; so, we know the things we should be eating.

Make a list of vegetables and what they resembles.

____

____

____

After getting gods prescription, in my head, it was really easy to give up donuts and soda. In the space provided jot down what a believer's diet should look like for one day.

____

____

____

____

____

Hosea 4:6 tells us that many people will die, because they do not have the knowledge. Hosea was talking about the first five books of scripture, because this is all the scripture they had at that time. The first five books of scripture laid out

God's design. If we want to live healthy we must eat healthy! The way we know how to eat is in God's guidelines.

To eat according to God's diet plan is life changing. I had to eliminate tons of food from my diet. It seems that I was being over filled. I was committing the sin of gluttony. The sin of gluttony has caused a major problem in America today. For example, obesity is almost the number one killer. Millions of dollars has been spent to help people learn the way they're supposed to eat and loose weight. Heart disease and diabetes is also a whole other issue in itself. Obesity, diabetes, and heart disease is not what God wanted for his people. He has called us out of the world. We are to resemble our creator and I don't think that our creator is going to be obese and sickly. In the space provided use your artistic ability to either draw or write down your thoughts about how the creator will look.

People today, both Christians and non-Christians, are not listening to the right knowledge. Yes, God put doctors here to help us, but some doctors hurt us instead. Doctors are trying to find the problem and provide medication. Our great physician not only diagnoses the problems, but He eliminates it. God does not give us a solution that will create another problem. God wants us to walk in health and wellness. He does not want us to suffer with sickness and disease. If you want to live a healthier life then perhaps we need to follow God's prescription. For me, it came down to the custom of men and my customs versus the Gods design.

The eating customs of mankind today, is to be so busy that we have no time to prepare fresh fruits and produce. Satan has distracted with all sorts of activities and resort going through the drive-through. We no longer have time to sit down to a meal together, talk about the day, and give advice to our children on how to solve their problems

appropriately. Satan has collided our need for

healthy living with distractions to keep us away

from what God has instructed for us to live.

____

____

____

____

____

____

Chapter 3: God's Time-Table.

In order to live a healthy life we must follow God's great design. We must lay aside the customs of mankind. The customs of mankind can be described as follows: eating often, eating too late, eating the wrong things, and consuming too much of everything. For example, I was guilty of going to a restaurant, sitting down to eat, and saying I was full, but when dessert came around I was ready to eat. The customs that I just mentioned above, including my example, are all forms of gluttony. (**Philippians 3:19** Whose end is destruction, whose God is their belly, and whose glory is in their shame, who mind earthly things.) Gluttony is a sin and Jesus said to go sin a no more. If Jesus said to go and sin no more then I had a decision to make and so do you! {**John 8:11** "She said, No man, LORD. And Jesus said unto her, Neither do I condemn thee: go, and sin no more."}

God created this world on his own time clock. Mankind has created their own time schedule to follow. The Bible says for us to eat the food when we see it. (**Exodus 16:12 and Exodus 12:8**) It is hard to see food in the night; therefore, we are not supposed to eat during the nighttime hours. If God was to make bananas, apples, and oranges in a neon color then perhaps that would tell us it was good to eat at night time. According to **Ecclesiastics 3:1**, there is a time and place that everything should occur. God's design is perfect and if we follow our creators design we will be healthy. For example, God made an orange; so that, we could grab it with our hands, peel it, break it open, and eat it. On the other hand, our creator made the tiger to run an extreme pace; therefore, we do not have the ability to chase it down and kill it with our bare hands. By design, we are not supposed to be eating Tigers.

God created 12 hours of daylight. Mankind decided to break God's plan and add minutes to create an hours. We are supposed to see our food and then eat our food, it makes sense that we only eat during the day. According to science, our bodies are made up of about 70% water and our body digest food better while we sleep. The organs work during the night to expel our food. Thus, I stopped eating late in the evening.   I did realize I was more hungry in the morning and wanted breakfast instead of a baked good item.

Scientists have also studied the moon extensively. In fact, we've even been there. The moon has a lot to do with our seasons. The seasons are controlled by the tides and some weather patterns. The moon and water has a definite correlation. Therefore, the moon tells us when we are supposed to stop eating and to sleep. It is not natural to stay up until midnight and eat late at night, because this repeated behavior causes problems with our health. For example, people have decided to make this their custom, the body started to rebel; so, we started going to the doctors. The doctors then, in return, decided to call our condition indigestion and started prescribing us a medication to take. Instead of going back to the Masters plan, Society in general decided to take the prescription, and continue with their custom. This custom is not natural; therefore, it begins to inhibit other body processes. When the body is not able to operate according to the Masters plan it causes more medical conditions.

Chapter 4: The box matters.

There are three boxes to consider when thinking about your health. The three boxes are as follows: the Television, the microwave, and the container in which your food is packaged. Today I would like for you to complete the following activity and then come back and finish your lesson.

One. When you watch television are you eating? If you are eating wow you are watching TV write down what you ate.

Two. If you use your microwave today record what you used it to cook.

Three. If you ate something frozen today write down what you eat and record how much calories, fat, protein, and sodium that was in the products.

Perhaps, one of the number one unhealthy customs society has today is eating while watching television. If we were all honest we could admit that we are partakers in this custom. Most dissed most of the time eating while watching TV is unnecessary eating. When I added up all of the calories I was consumed during watching TV I was amazed. I began making it a rule not to eat while watching TV and I began to lose a few ounces a week. Then, I discovered I needed to have my hands doing something; so, I begin making cards and scarves. Finally, turn the TV off and I picked up my Bible and began to study and right. The television box is One societies major unhealthy custom today.

The microwave is also one of America's unhealthy habits also. If we do not finish our meals they can be easily warmed up in the microwave box; so that, we can sit down in front of the television box and continue in our gluttonous ways. Did you know; that if you warm water up in the microwave and feed it to your plant that it will die.? Yes there's some kind of process some kind of chemicals that the microwave gives off that actually kills gods vegetation. My question is if water warmed in the microwave kills gods plants then what does my microwavable food due to my body when I consume it?

The third box, which also is a custom, but I would like to mention is the TV dinner. There are currently hundreds TV dinners that we can buy in the frozen section of the grocery store. Some of them are even considered to be a healthy option, But are they really? After what we've learned about the plant dying; I would say that a boxed TV dinner is one of the worst things that we could consume. I challenge you to find your most favorite TV dinner and prepare it your self. Notice the taste difference and then notice the calories and sodium you have consumed. Which one is truly healthy for you? Following God's diet plan will make us healthy from the inside out.

Because God created the vegetation of the world we should eat lots of fruits and vegetables. So I'm dietitian to say 50% of your diet should be fruits and vegetables. We should be consuming at least one green leafy plant a day, Because those plants contain chlorophyll. Chlorophyll in The body helps clean the blood. My favorite leafy vegetable would be spinach. I like to put spinach in my egg omelets in the morning. I like lettuce in my salad for lunch. I also like to make kale chips in the oven from fresh kale. Steamed broccoli can be added to any mail. God created everything for a reason. For example, my favorite horse, whose name was freedom, was fed correctly, but freedom had a sweet sweet tooth as well. His sweet tooth often caused him to be constipated and he did not like how we had to clean him out. This same principle we can add to our own bodies. If we do not put in our bodies what God tells us to put in it;

then, we are going to get sick.

Chapter Five: Our customs are not always what's best for us!

The customs that society has today are very anti-Christ or opposite of what Christ desires for us to enjoy today. Learning what God wants for us is always what is best for us. I have been on several diet and I have had some success, that old habits and bad customs have creeped back into my life resulting in weight gain. Truly understanding that God requires us to walk in health and wellness has help me keep the weight off, because God diet plan ears the best for everyone.

God is the creator of all things and he knows all things. For example John 1:1 tells us that he was the word and is the word. God created all creeping things, buzzing things flying file, And he knows

how they operate. He knows what comes in and

out of every been on earth. For example, I know

we would agree that God created our bodies and he

created them flawless. He knows what it takes to

run our bodies and he knows what it takes to ruin

our bodies. Let's review the law of Moses. And the

chart below generate a list of what we should eat

and what we should not eat. Scripture informs us

that what we should eat is called clean and what

we should not eat is called unclean.

Clean	Unclean

Leviticus 11:9-12. These shall ye eat of all that are in the waters: whatsoever hath fins and scales in the waters, in the seas, and in the rivers, them shall ye eat. 10And all that have not fins and scales in the seas, and in the rivers, of all that move in the waters, and of any living thing which is in the

waters, they shall be an abomination unto you:

11They shall be even an abomination unto you; ye shall not eat of their flesh, but ye shall have their carcases in abomination. 12Whatsoever hath no fins nor scales in the waters, that shall be an abomination unto you.

Deuteronomy 14:3-20 King James Version (KJV)

3 Thou shalt not eat any abominable thing.

4 These are the beasts which ye shall eat: the ox, the sheep, and the goat,

5 The hart, and the roebuck, and the fallow deer, and the wild goat, and the pygarg, and the wild ox, and the chamois.

6 And every beast that parteth the hoof, and cleaveth the cleft into two claws, and cheweth the cud among the beasts, that ye shall eat.

7 Nevertheless these ye shall not eat of them that chew the cud, or of them that divide the cloven hoof; as the camel, and the hare, and the coney: for they chew the cud, but divide not the hoof; therefore they are unclean unto you.

8 And the swine, because it divideth the hoof, yet cheweth not the cud, it is unclean unto you: ye shall not eat of their flesh, nor touch their dead carcase.

9 These ye shall eat of all that are in the waters: all that have fins and scales shall ye eat:

10 And whatsoever hath not fins and scales ye may not eat; it is unclean unto you.

11 Of all clean birds ye shall eat.

12 But these are they of which ye shall not eat: the eagle, and the ossifrage, and the ospray,

13 And the glede, and the kite, and the vulture after his kind,

14 And every raven after his kind,

15 And the owl, and the night hawk, and the cuckow, and the hawk after his kind,

16 The little owl, and the great owl, and the swan,

17 And the pelican, and the gier eagle, and the cormorant,

18 And the stork, and the heron after her kind, and

the lapwing, and the bat.

19 And every creeping thing that flieth is unclean

unto you: they shall not be eaten.

20 But of all clean fowls ye may eat.

Leviticus 11 Eating – or touching the carcass of –

any seafood without fins or scales (11:10-12)

1.   Eating – or touching the carcass of – eagle, the

vulture, the black vulture, the red kite, any kind of

black kite, any kind of raven, the horned owl, the

screech owl, the gull, any kind of hawk, the little

owl, the cormorant, the great owl, the white owl,

the desert owl, the osprey, the stork, any kind of

heron, the hoopoe and the bat. (11:13-19)

2.   Eating – or touching the carcass of – flying

insects with four legs, unless those legs are jointed

(11:20-22)

3.   Eating any animal which walks on all four and

has paws (11:27)

4.   Eating – or touching the carcass of – the

weasel, the rat, any kind of great lizard, the gecko,

the monitor lizard, the wall lizard, the skink and

the chameleon (11:29)

5. Eating an animal which doesn't both chew cud

and has a divided hoof (cf: camel, rabbit, pig)

(11:4-7)

Chapter Six: Did the new covenant really say we could eat anything we set our eyes upon?

Matthew 1:22 informs us that Jesus came not to do away with the law but just to fulfill it. Jesus fulfilled all types of prophecy recorded in the Old Testament. Continue reading the book of Matthew and when you get to chapter 5 about verse 18 Jesus tells us to keep the laws. Jesus explains that not one jot or tittle of the scripture shall be changed as long as heaven and Earth is sustaining.

Peter had a dream in Acts chapter 10 and many Bible scholars suggests that this dream means that it is ok for mankind to consume anything they wish. However, this dream is not really discussing what we physically are to consume. Peter knew

Jesus very well and trusted him. He submitted himself to Jesus and to the gospel. He knew all the laws as they were written and he knew what was clean and unclean to eat. This dream took place three times and he said that he had never eaten anything and clean; which, he pondered the meaning of the vision. Peter questions God in versus 16, 17, and 18 about the meaning of the vision. As time passed Peter grew uneasy and was uncertain about the interpretation of the dream, because he followed the customs of the Jews.

According to **Acts 10:8-10** God was not talking about eating unclean creatures. In the space provided read Acts 10:8-10 and write down what his dream was to teach us.

____

____

____

____

____

We are in fact sinning when we enjoy our customs of eating, because oftentimes the customs are totally opposite from what God has told us we can consume. For example, in **Acts 10:27-28** Peter made the trip to Cornelius's house there was many people gathered. The issue of the group was that the religious leaders of the Jews had a law that stated Jews could have no association with the outside world and God was telling Peter that this was wrong, because through Jesus Christ God made everyone clean. The fact that we are all cleansed through the blood of Jesus Christ and are washed in baptism is the requirement that makes us adopted sons and daughters of God. Who are we to differentiate the difference between God's children? God has to set free both bond, free, man, and woman and all of us are on a level playing field. Therefore, it is evil in the sight of the Lord to call any man or woman unclean or common. Thanks be to Jesus that we are all joint heirs with him and that we are royalty.

Chapter 7: Can we eat anything as long as we bless it?

Blessing our food can be as simple as thanking God for it! We usually bless our food by saying prayer before we eat our food. First Timothy 4:3 does not give us the permission to eat anything as long as we pray over it. God told us certain things were for food and the other things that we consume are not food. According to his scripture we are told to eat what is good.

So, what is good to eat? What does good mean according to Scripture? To find the answer to the posing questions let's examine the creation story and the account of Noah. In Genesis, God created the world in six days and rested on the seventh. He called his creation good. Therefore, all of God's creation is good including His decrees. In addition, God told Noah to take seven of each of the clean animals and only two of the unclean animals.

Chapter 8: Description of Romans 12

Romans 12 explains to us that we are holy temples and we are supposed to obey God as our reasonable service. We think of our church as a temple and we care a great deal about what goes in and comes out of that temple. For this reason we should care about what goes in our body. In addition, most people know the scripture where God said it's not what goes into the temple that defiles the temple but it's what comes out of a person that defiles them, but God also said we should only put in our temple things that he has blessed. Finally, as far as our food is concerned, if we put good nutrition in our bodies then we will become more healthy.

Some of the most reliable preachers and teachers have taught me that you may eat whatever you want as long as you ask God for his blessing and thank him for it; however, this is not a teaching from the New Testament. I believe this teaching is one of societies customs, because the New Testament does not teach us about what is considered to be food.

The Torah has been rejected by most Christian denominations today and is not taught effectively. We get our instruction about how to eat from the following chapters in the Bible: Genesis, Leviticus, and Deuteronomy. It seems that people decide what they think is food according to what tastes good to them. Most people decide that food is

consumable if it tastes great. Jesus even warned us
about listening to the scribes, the Pharisees, the
religious leaders, and the government, because
what we see today is them defining what is food.
Don't we have the FDA?

Chapter 9: Why should we not consume herbs; such as, marijuana?

The Bible is God's word and is our instruction book for life. We must not miss use it, because this would cause us to go astray. For example, the use of marijuana for health reasons is perhaps what God created marijuana for, but using marijuana for recreational purposes goes against what God requires for each one of us. Consider Ephesians 5:18, because it explains to us that Christians should be sober-minded. We should not drink to get drunk and we should not use drugs to alter the state of our mind or being.

God requires his children to walk just and up right. We are to be vigilant and ready to respond to

God's voice at all times. If we are walking in an altered state of mind we are in capable of meeting God's requirement. Finally, Jesus's blood to freely given on the cross, this has given us a new life and made us a new creature and we are cleansed. Therefore, we are supposed to be mindful of our actions and obedient to God's statutes.

Consider what Paul instructs us in the matter of judging others by reading Colossians 2:14. What does this scripture and the Holy Spirit tell you about living under grace? Remember, to consider the last paragraph we just discussed.

Leviticus 11:9 through 12.

Deuteronomy 14

Leviticus six the priests and offerings

Chapter 10: should we all be vegans?

According to this scripture God's people are supposed to eat meat. In fact, the priests ate very well. God said that this was not a an abomination, but a way to provide for his servants. The priest were to take oil and flower and add it to the meet; which, could perhaps have been a country fried steak. Protein is needed in our bodies to make it work affectively. Proteins make our muscles work and gives us a pretty appearance, because the minerals help create strong teeth and hair follicles.

According to Genesis chapter 18 there was a man named Abraham. The angel of the Lord appeared to Abraham. Some biblical scholars think that this was Jesus Christ incarnated. According to this account, the Lord and to Angels showed up in front of Abraham during the middle of the day. Abraham made the men comfortable under a tree and then went to Sarah. Sarah made cakes for the men; meanwhile, Abraham killed a cow and offered it to the Lord and the two angels. In addition, in Jesus's ministry he sat with many people and ate meat. Jesus meat with a great multitude! Remember, He fed them with the seven loaves of bread and two fishes. Moreover, in John chapter 21 the Lord Jesus told them to cast their nets on the other side and they caught a great multitude of fish to eat. Finally, and Luke 22:8 Jesus ate Passover dinner which was lamb.

Chapter 11: Are Christians permitted to consume sacrificed to idols?

First Timothy 1:1-5 Sustain from meat. The Catholics.

First Corinthian's chapter 8 don't offend your brother by eating meat

Romans 14 also deals with meat sacrificed to other gods

One of the battles in the initial church was disturbed by how meat; which, had been sacrificed to idols was being consumed by New Christians. Today, I would not eat anything that was sacrificed to idols! So, these debates over what to eat was debated over long ago and still is a concern in our modern society. To first-century new converts if they sat down and ate the meant to idols they could have suffered great consequence. As the apostles dealt with the issue! These apostles gave directions on selected topics. These topics and directions still provide Christians today's with application processes.

In the initial times of the church both the Gentiles and Jewish believers were in fellowship with each other. An issue arose concerning the eating of meat, because the Greco-Roman society was rooted with idol worship. Therefore, in the marketplace sold meats that had been sacrificed to their false gods. The Jews understood this meat to be unclean. The gentiles was concerned with the food-handling practices of the non-Christians.

Eating of the consecrated meat was also concerned to be a "second-hand" idolatry. Today, I stopped selling my goats, because I discovered that men were both driving long distances, to buy my white goats; so, they could sacrifice them to their god's.

The church in Syrian Antioch, consist of of both Jews and Gentiles. Their struggle with eating meat sacrificed to idols was a real issue (**Acts 15**). The Jerusalem Council had the last word! They decided to urge the Gentile converts to refrain from food and substances sacrificed to idols (**Acts 15:29**). We should all obey the principle of self-denial. All Christians should be eager to put aside their personal desires to maintain unity in the body of Christ. Finally, the spiritual growth of other members should have importance over individual inclinations.

In **1 Corinthians 8:4-13**, Paul further explains this subject. Paul stated that eating meat offered to an idol was not immoral. He described food as not an avenue to bring us near to God. When it comes to this matter, it seams that it does not matter if we eat meat. However, Paul impresses on the hearts of the believer that under no circumstances, should we encourage another person to violate their conscience. Titus 1:15 discusses the issue of purity! Therefore, it is clear that one should never to eat meat again if it would cause "A Child of God" to transgress against their own conscience.

Chapter 12: God's wisdom is light! Let's be beacons!

Focus scriptures Ephesians 5:1- & Daniel 12:3

Ephesians 5:8-9 8For ye were sometimes darkness, but now are ye light in the LORD: walk as children of light: 9(For the fruit of the Spirit is in all goodness and righteousness and truth;)

Daniel 12:3

Those who are wise shall shine

Like the brightness of the firmament,

And those who turn many to righteousness

Like the stars forever and ever.

When we study and meditate on the Scriptures of the Bible we grow in godly wisdom. That ideas and concepts that we usually do not understand we'll suddenly make sense, because the Holy Spirit will teach them to us. Sometimes, the solutions to our crazy problems will become clear. The only way to gain a clear understanding is to become beacons of wisdom. For example, the word of God brightens our understanding and other folks should be able to witness that understanding in us. People should be able to see what that we belong to the Lord.

Challenge one: After examining the events that took place this last year use the space provided to generate a list of how your thoughts, ideas, attitudes, and actions have changed into being more Christlike.

This next year my next step comes in the form of a New Year's resolution is to become more Christlike and to be healthy inside and out. I desire Godly wisdom to look and act different. I want to obey God and live separate from the world. If you have a similar goal check out my healthy believers group on Facebook. We are going to allow God's word to cleanse us inside and out.

One way to experience good Christian advice is to follow any visions chapter 5. Please read this passage and it's entirety. I have been as Paul advised in this chapter has great rewards. In the space provided list 10 statements that describes Paul's advice.

1. _____________________________

____

____

2. _____________________________

____

____

3.

____

____

____

4. ____

____

____

5. ____

____

____

6. ____

____

____

7. ____

____

8. ______________________________

____

____

9. ______________________________

____

10.______________________________

____

____

The Holy Spirit explains that if we are
Christians we should live good lives. For example,
in verses one and two it's clear that we should
imitate the reactions of God if we are his children.
According to verse four, Paul reminds us to use
clean speech, because what comes out of our
mouth is a reflection of what's in our soul.

Christian speech reflects the goodness of God and may draw mankind to him. However if we do not imitate God and have clean healthy speech we'll do the opposite for mankind. Dirty speech drawls mankind to sin not to godliness.

At this time, please re-read verses five through 17. Notice how believers are supposed to respond to nonbelievers. Where is Christian should become friends with nonbelievers for the purpose of drawling them into the light, but we must be careful that we Listen and follow the instructions of the Holy Spirit, because Santa is Tim Dana and we may come involved in it. Christians should have actions that reflect our face. We should skip stain from evil pleasures and even flee from dangerous and evil conditions. So, we do not slip

in to sin because sin will take us further than we

want to go.

Christians must know the expectations of God

and follow them. And passages 18 through 20 we

learned that God expects this from us. Paul asks us

to look at how alcohol affects a drunk and explains

that are confessions should follow the Holy Spirit

in the same manner. Finally, in passage 20 we find

another antidote to depression. We can infer that

when depression hits that we should meditate on

the blessings that we have received, because this

makes the melancholy Spirit flea. The love of God

ensures our strength.

The word of God shines a light through this wicked world; so, we can see without tripping! Following the advice of the Bible will cause us to become more Christlike. Our stumbles will lead us to the perfect flight. Consider the meaning of the following scriptures: **Psalms 119:130 and Psalm 119:105.** With the word of God we see clearly and we do have to risk tripping over the huge ruts life can bring. For example, in our scriptural reading for today Ephesians 5 we are the light of the world. If we have the light of Jesus inside us; then, we can be a beacon of light that shines through the darkness of this world.

As this new year begins log onto Facebook and join our Facebook group: healthy believers. As we grow in Christ He grants us wisdom. Being in a group of people who seek Christ will be beneficial, because we can provide godly counsel for one another. Let's all be stars of God's wisdom. Let's be a people that other seek out for prayer and gardens. The wisdom of God provides will help you shine; so, you can help others on their way. This light will also lead others to Christ for repentance and forgiveness. Below I have included included one of my favorite scriptures and in the space provided you may jot down its meaning **Proverbs 4:7-9!**

____

____

____

Proverbs 4:7-9 7Wisdom is the principal thing; therefore get wisdom: and with all thy getting get understanding. 8Exalt her, and she shall promote thee: she shall bring thee to honour, when thou dost embrace her. 9She shall give to thine head an ornament of grace: a crown of glory shall she deliver to thee.

This Scripture describes wisdom as an ornament of grace. This ornament grants us grace and glory, but it also points to Jesus.

Chapter 14: Your Body is the Holy Temple

Have you ever meditated on the look and feel of the Holy Temple? If so, then you know how special we are to God! It is beautiful to know that we are the Holy Temple. When I think about the Holy Temple I image gold, silver, costly gems, and the finer things of life, but really the first temples we read about in scripture were built to be the dwelling place of God. However, today the only thing we have to offer God is our fleshly bodies. Let's face it, some of us take better care of the Holy Temple than others. Nevertheless, God prefers our fleshly bodies over gold, silver, and wealth!

For today's Bible study let's read **1 Corinthians 6:1-20**! Focus on 1 Corinthians 6:19, because it reads: **"1 Corinthians 6:19**(KJV) "19 What? know ye not that your body is the temple of the Holy Ghost which is in you, which ye have of God, and ye are not your own?" Then, the message of this scripture is echoed in **Romans 12:**1; which states: "12 I beseech you therefore, brethren, by the mercies of God, that ye present your bodies a living sacrifice, holy, acceptable unto God, which is your reasonable service."

Our bodies are not only the Temple that Houses the Lord, but they are also a living sacrifice! In the days of the Old Testament, the father of each family would have to travel to the Temple and bring their best sacrifice. Sometimes, it was a mile

or two; while, for others it may have meant days of

travel. Thankyou God, that the ultimate sacrifice

for sin was paid through Jesus Christ, The spotless

Lamb of God, and there is no more sacrifice of

lambs and bulls. Under the New Covenant, we

give sacrifices to God from the fruit of our lips.

We lay aside lusts, selfish desires, and personal

goals to perform Godly tasks. For example, what

examples does **Hebrews 13:1** present as our praise

for God resembles?

____

____

____

We all realize that welcoming God into our hearts and asking Him to forgive us of our sin is a good thing, but many times we miss the part of where we are to give Him complete control over our lives. When we give ourselves completely to God, inside and out, a deep void in our soul is filled. Allowing God to have complete control over our lives relinquishes many of lives problems and quenches a lot of the fiery darts of Satanic power.

Today, would you give every part of your life to God especially if you have not done so in the past? Please consider, **1 Corinthians 6:20** (KJV)

"20 For ye are bought with a price: therefore glorify God in your body, and in your spirit, which are God's"

Chapter 13: How do we overcome obstacles and be victorious?

We need to overcome the obstacles in our life by abiding in the vine. Jesus Christ is the vine! Our goal, according to scripture, is to abide in the vine and bear much fruit for the kingdom of God. Some people believe that bearing fruit is their imprint left behind for mankind or the belongings they acquire during their life is their fruit, but nothing could be further from the truth. Let's consider Johns writings in chapter 15 and focus first on John 15:5.

John 15:5 I am the vine, ye are the branches: He that abideth in me, and I in him, the same bringeth forth much fruit: for without me ye can do nothing.

John explains that our lives are only productive after we receive salvation. Through the teaching of John it becomes perfectly clear of how much we need Jesus. Curiously, John echoes what Jesus also taught us in John 6. Jesus taught us that He was also the bread of life. Remarkably, the lecture on The Bread of Life occurred fairly early in the ministry of Jesus; while, this writing by John, occurred at the end of Jesus's ministry. Jesus's seminar, here in John, occurred while speaking to His disciples, after His final Passover observance. Jesus explained that our vines cannot produce fruit apart from Christ. This segment of scripture leaves the impression that we are to make every effort to remain "in" Him, not permitting what just transpired with Judas happen to us. Juda betrayed

His Savior. Judas deserted his accountability enforced by the New Covenant.

What is the fruit that comes from the vines of Jesus? (We are the branches of Jesus)

____

____

____

____

In the language of the Greek, the word fruit is described as, "karpos." Obviously, Karpos denotes that the fruit comes from vines or trees. In the Old Testament, the fruit also referred to the children which were born in the family. However, in the New Testament, bearing fruit for the Christians, specifically means producing similar attributes of the tree. For example, God created a grape vine to produce grapes; therefore, the vine produces grapes and not lemons. As for the Christian, the fruit that is born is similar to the nature and quality of the plant from which it came from and some of that fruit is found in, **Galatians 5:22-25**.

Galatians 5 reads: "22But the fruit of the Spirit is love, joy, peace, forbearance, kindness, goodness, faithfulness, 23gentleness and self-control. Against such things there is no law. 24Those who belong to Christ Jesus have crucified the flesh with its passions and desires. 25Since we live by the Spirit, let us keep in step with the Spirit."

The key to Jesus's teaching is that the fruit we bear is a type, a quality, and a substance of which is becoming of Christ. The spiritual fruit does not come from the flesh. The fruit is produced through our flesh by the Holy Spirit!

Part 2: How do we abide in Christ?

To abide in Christ means to remain and dwell. This is where we live! The word abode means to set up a residence or habitation of a place where you will live. Christ wants to live inside of us! If Jesus lives inside of us then we will have some of His attributes. These attributes when nourish flow out of our being and produce fruit. First, John 14:6 states that Jesus is the way, the truth, and the life, but scripture also states that Jesus walked walk in peace, truth, love, and forgiveness. Therefore in

the following scriptures note the attributes of Jesus
Christ.

Isa. 9:6

____

Romans 8:39

____

1 John 4:7-8

____

John 1:1

____

John 1:14

____

Therefore, we choose to walk in love, peace,
truth, and forgiveness, we are abiding in the Lord.

When we walk in the counsel of scripture, we become wise, and we are abiding in Christ(making our house) in the Glory of God. Finally, when we do this we are living in the vine. Thus, receiving the best nourishment for our branches. We will see the fruits of salvation for our families, healings, miracles, and all the promises of scriptures will be fulfilled before our very eyes.

Part 3: The symbolism of The Bread of Life and The fruit of the vine.

For another moment, consider the beginning of our relationship with Christ! We can't overlook the gospel (Jesus birth, death, and resurrection). Jesus paid the penalty for our sins and without him there would be no future for us except for death and the second death. Without our savior, Jesus Christ, there would be no yearning for the Kingdom of God. In fact, Jesus made it possible for us to be the vine and through Him we can bear fruit for the kingdom. Understanding this symbolism and mystery of scripture we can grasp how much we need and what Christ did for us. To glean as much as we can from this text, we need to connect our learning with Jesus's final Passover, because Jesus introduced the idea the He was the bread of life as a Passover symbol. This symbolism in scripture connect us to why we should conduct communion. For example, Paul writes in **I Corinthians 11:23-24:** "For I received from the Lord that which I also delivered to you: that the Lord Jesus on the same night in which He was betrayed took bread; and when He had given thanks, He broke it and said, "Take eat; this is My body which is broken for you; do this in remembrance of Me."

According to John 6, bread plays an important role in conveying the message Christ wants us to receive. This message frequently used as a metaphor for Christ Himself. These symbols are important to grasping what Christ teaches in John 15:1-6. The vine, Christ's speaks of is obviously the grape vine. He clearly states that He is the vine and that we are the branches attached to Him. Just as the grapes, in our example, can be produced only by a shoot that remains attached to the vine, we can only produce spiritual fruit that pleases the

Father. In this message, all nourishment that results in fruit must come from the vine. Jesus not only pays the penalty of our sins, but He also supplies the spiritual nourishment that produces fruit; which, glorifies the Father and prepares us for life in God's Kingdom.

Part 4: Conclusion

To end today's message, please consider what John wrote in chapter 8. **John 8:31-32** { 31Then said Jesus to those Jews which believed on him, If ye continue in my word, then are ye my disciples indeed; 32And ye shall know the truth, and the truth shall make you free.} reminds us that continuing in God's Word is the key to knowing the truth and becoming free. This greatly enhances the production of fruit. Thus, if we fulfill our responsibility, we can in essence be partakers in a partnership with Jesus. In this partnership we will have influence over the evilness that exists in the world. With such a partnership in Jesus Christs we will Remaining in Him, and this is the only way we will faithfully fulfill their roles generated by God for our lives. Finally, after fulfilling our Earthly callings we will be called up to Heaven where we will remain for eternality.

Chapter 13: Is our food contaminated?

One of my main goals, since all of my mini strokes, has been to regain mental status. In order to understand God's word and to teach about God's word I must have an ability to learn, to understand, to memorize, and to explain. Have been actively seeking God to restore these things to me. However, the little voice inside my conscience has been instructing me to learn about health and wellness. That still small voice inside my soul has been encouraging me to lose weight. I have determined that if God made or created it for food then eat it, but if man has made something and call it food then I should leave it. For example, God did not make a Twinkie. In fact, The Twinkie is shaped like a coffin. If we consume too many

Twinkies and then we will end up in a coffin.

Many doctors and dietitians (researchers at

George Washington University) have discovered

that artificial flavorings are not good for us.

Artificial flavorings can cause high blood sugar,

High blood pressure, high cholesterol, and

abdominal fat. Our Bible tells us that if we need

something sweet to eat honey, cinnamon, and fresh

fruit. One reason we have these artificial flavorings

and we are addicted to them is, because they were

created based on poor science. Another example of

poor science is cloning animals for consumption.

Our government could make a substantial amount

of money from this cologne meet; therefore, they

will obtain many well-known scientists to present it to the public. These scientists would tell us that there has been no lasting effects of the meat. However, since the 60s and 70s cancer is ramp it and other illnesses have caused many deaths.

Next, consider the words of **Ezekiel 4:13**! (Ezekiel 4:13 13And the LORD said, Even thus shall the children of Israel eat their defiled bread among the Gentiles, whither I will drive them.) This scripture warns us that in the last days our food will not be good for us. For example, the United States government has known since the 1960s that our food sources are not substantial enough to feed America. We do not have enough grassland to feed the animals; therefore we do not have enough animals. Perhaps, this is why the government decided to genetically modify our food. Genetic modification could perhaps be explained as genetic mutation. For example, the government is a business. The government cares more about money than it does it's own people. The government does not care about our health or if we become extinct, because we are already over populated. The government has created a genetically modified tree, because there has been AN increase in demand for wood. The government can now grow a pine tree in three years. Then, they harvest the tree and make wood, but a major problem with this is that piece of wood can break in half by stomping on it. If they genetically modified tree is not worth buying them why do we think genetically modified food is OK?

Consider the food and and drug administration. How is it ran? Well basically, the farmers pay the organization big bucks to promote their foods. This organization works for the government to regulate America's food, but it makes a large profit from it! Dr. Highman at Cleveland clinic; which is a dietary specialist, told me that the food pyramid given to us from the government should be called the coffin, because these guidelines do nothing, but line the pockets of government officials. Another example to be concerned the FDA recommends a cup of coffee every morning is good for you. My friend, coffee is not my enemy, the caffeine is my enemy.

Caffeine is a drug and it is also found in most of

our soft drinks. The consumption of products like

Pepsi or Coca-Cola will calls you to become

aesthetic. Wants, I witnessed a science project at

school. The experiment part of this project

consisted of one cup of Pepsi, 1 cup of Coca-Cola,

and two dimes. There was enough acid in the soft

drinks two calls the dams to Sean. Brothers and

sisters if we are drinking soda pop then we are

consuming pure acid. In addition, The properties

within caffeine bring you up, but then you fall.

This is the same thing that some street level drugs

do for folks. Corporate America is addicted to

caffeine, but most people I know are also addicted

to caffeine. This perhaps is what our government

wanted for the people, because now that we are addicted to the officials can place an extra tax on the merchandise. In the morning or throughout the day when we crave a caffeine we should actually do some type of exercise. God created our bodies to move. God gave us nutritional guidelines to follow not to restrict us, but to help us maintain efficient bodily movements. If we are sick we cannot serve God like he designed. **Mark 16:16** gives us the great commission for gods children. In the space provided, record what God commands each of us to fulfill.

Chapter 14 God promises us prosperity!

Do you believe that whatever you do will prosper? This year, how can we cash in on that promise? In one of our last lesson we discussed how important prayer is in our lives. In fact, we discussed how to become prayer warrior. Today, let's examine how we can make this dream statement mean something in our lives. Consider what psalm 1:3 states.

Psalm 1-3 King James Version (KJV)

1 Blessed is the man that walketh not in the counsel of the ungodly, nor standeth in the way of sinners, nor sitteth in the seat of the scornful.

2 But his delight is in the law of the Lord; and in his law doth he meditate day and night.

3 And he shall be like a tree planted by the rivers of water, that bringeth forth his fruit in his season; his leaf also shall not wither; and whatsoever he doeth shall prosper.

A person is blessed to work for sake in all that God. God doesn't care about our race or gender, because he created us all in his image. The writer of this psalm states that those who obey God or like healthy, fruit bearing trees, with strong roots in the word. Then, the way of the disobedient is rebellion and death. Beginning in verse for the author changes sides a bit. continue reading **Psalm 1:4-7.**

4 The ungodly are not so: but are like the chaff which the wind driveth away.

5 Therefore the ungodly shall not stand in the judgment, nor sinners in the congregation of the righteous.

6 For the Lord knoweth the way of the righteous: but the way of the ungodly shall perish.

The author describes how joyous it is when we obey God, but when we have friends or relationships that go against God, sometimes we begin to sin, because we do not oppose their ways in their views. Friends need to have common ground in which to stand on, friends against God brings oppression and sadness don't Lord.

There is power in praying the word of God over ourselves and our love ones. Consider first Corinthian's chapter 3.

1 Corinthians 3:6-7 King James Version (KJV)

6 I have planted, Apollos watered; but God gave the increase.

7 So then neither is he that planteth any thing, neither he that watereth; but God that giveth the increase.

Paul continually prayed, but did not take all the credit for people being saved, because he also mentioned Apollo as a minister hard at work. Just because we are in prayer about one particular person in one particular situation does not mean that God answered our prayers alone. "It takes a village to raise a child", have you heard of that expression? Well, that's the same principle here! One person prays, the next person Added to the situation, and God gives the increase to the kingdom. Prayer warriors are therefore needed in the body of Christ.

Let's practice praying for I love one to be stronger and better match fruit for the Lord. Turn back with me to some one and replace the word key with your name or a name of a friend. I'll use my daughter Elaina, because she will soon be off to college. Lord, I thank you, that you have blessed Elaina. Allow her walk, stand, or sit with ungodly and scornful. Let her delight in your law; while, meditating on your word day and night. Allow her to be like a tree, you planted, by the rivers that brings good fruit. Let her spiritual gifts John and not with her. Allow her Cummings and her goings to prosper beauty for the kingdom. Amen!

Finally, I would like for you to turn with me to Proverbs 15 and let's read the verses one through four.

Proverbs 15:1-4 King James Version (KJV)

15 A soft answer turneth away wrath: but grievous words stir up anger.

2 The tongue of the wise useth knowledge aright: but the mouth of fools poureth out foolishness.

3 The eyes of the Lord are in every place, beholding the evil and the good.

4 A wholesome tongue is a tree of life: but perverseness therein is a breach in the spirit

As Christians we should all want to be ministers of wisdom and healing. This scripture describes how we should use our words. We should be at tree of life that breathes goodness and mercy. However, if we are not careful with our speech we can breach the spirit. we can be contrary to the word of God. **Proverbs 18:21** explains that we can create death with our tongue (speech).

Proverbs 18:21 King James Version

21 Death and life are in the power of the tongue: and they that love it shall eat the fruit thereof

I love to proclaim the scriptures over my children. So, let's practice! If you do not have a child use your name. Oh, Lord! I'm grateful that Juliana's tongue is the tree of life. Help her speak the words of health and wisdom. Let her be a tree planted by the rivers that will bring forth good and plentiful fruit. Allow her gifts to shine and not wither. Allow, her to prosper and declare the name of the Lord. Amen!

using the powerful words of God in our prayers will invoke a reaction from God. He is faithful and just to hear an answer his children. The good news is that we are all children of God and what He promises is coming true. Continuing to use scripture in our prayer life will make us prayer warriors and it will make miracles happen.

Chapter 15: Delicious Traditional Jewish Cuisine.

Recipe One: Hamantaschen

This dessert signifies, to many celebrants means, the shape of the triangular hat supposedly worn by Haman, the villain of the story in the Book of Esther. However, there's more history than that to the cookie — and clues can be found in its name. For example, food critics state the idea of naming a pastry after someone "wicked" is to "turn it into something sweet,"

Ingredients:

3 eggs
1 cup granulated sugar
C&H Pure Cane Granulated Sugar 4 Lb

3/4 cup vegetable oil

2 1/2 teaspoons vanilla extract

1/2 cup orange juice

Tropicana Pure Premium No Pulp 100% Original Orange Juice 59 Fl Oz

5 1/2 cups all-purpose flour

1 tablespoon baking powder

1 cup fruit preserves, any flavor

Preheat oven to 350 degrees F (175 degrees C).

Grease cookie sheets.

In a large bowl, beat the eggs and sugar until

lightly and fluffy. Stir in the oil, vanilla and orange

juice. Combine the flour and baking powder; stir

into the batter to form a stiff dough. If dough is not

stiff enough to roll out, stir in more flour. On a

lightly floured surface, roll dough out to 1/4 inch

in thickness. Cut into circles using a cookie cutter

or the rim or a drinking glass. Place cookies 2

inches apart onto the prepared cookie sheets.

Spoon about 2 teaspoons of preserves into the

center of each one. Pinch the edges to form three

corners.

Bake for 12 to 15 minutes in the preheated oven,

or until lightly browned. Allow cookies to cool for

1 minute on the cookie sheet before removing to

wire racks to cool completely.

Per Serving: 246 calories; 7.7 g fat; 40 g

carbohydrates; 3.8 g protein; 23 mg cholesterol; 56

mg sodium.

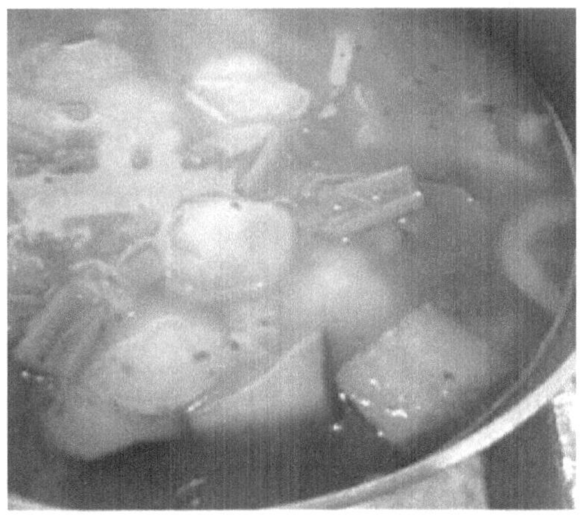

You might also like Recipe Two:

Matzo Soup Balls

"A great and tasty traditional meal. Serve in a soup, or in a bowl of milk. Either way it's great!! This is an old family recipe. I hope you will enjoy it as much as I have every Christmas and Hanukkah morning!" It was originally called Knedelack wich is Yiddush for dumpling.

Comes from:
https://www.allrecipes.com/recipe/37068/matzo-balls/?internalSource=hub%20recipe&referringContentTyp e=Search&clickId=cardslot%201

Ingredients

3 tablespoons pareve margarine, melted

2 eggs

1 cup matzo meal

1/2 teaspoon salt

Great Value Salt, 26 oz

1/2 cup water, or as needed

Directions:

In a medium bowl, whisk together the margarine and eggs until well blended. Combine the matzo meal and salt; lightly stir into the egg mixture until the liquid is absorbed, and the meal is damp. Gradually mix in the water so that the mixture holds together, but is not too wet. Cover and refrigerate while bringing the water to a boil.

Bring a large pot of lightly salted water to a boil. When the water is at a full boil, remove the matzo mixture from the refrigerator. Using wet hands, shape spoonfuls of the dough into balls. Do

not pack the balls together too tightly.

Drop balls into the boiling water, and boil

for 15 minutes. Remove from water and serve in

soup or cold milk. Do not let the matzo balls sit out

too long, or they will harden.

Nutrition Facts

**Per Serving: 127 calories; 6.1 g fat; 15.6 g
carbohydrates; 3.6 g protein; 53 mg cholesterol;
241 mg sodium.**

Recipe three: SHAKSHUKA (Breakfast)

"Try this tasty keto and paleo breakfast shakshuka full of greens! Delicious, quick, and so easy to make in just minutes in your Instant Pot®!"This is served in a hot dish.

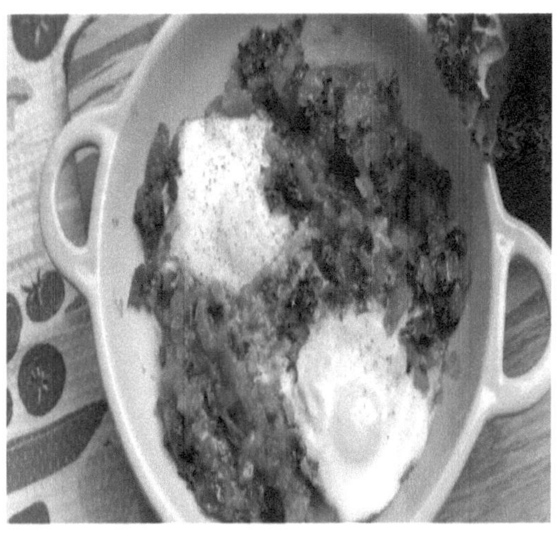

Ingredients:

1 tablespoon olive oil

1/2 onion, diced

1/2 red bell pepper, diced

2 cloves garlic, minced

1 teaspoon chili powder

1/2 teaspoon smoked paprika

1/2 teaspoon ground cumin

2 cups baby kale

1 1/2 cups marinara sauce

1/2 teaspoon sea salt

1/2 teaspoon ground black pepper

4 eggs

Brown Eggs 12 Ct

1 tablespoon chopped fresh parsley

Ready In 30 m

Turn on a multi-functional pressure cooker

(such as Instant Pot(R)) and select Saute function.

Heat olive oil and cook onion, red bell pepper,

garlic, chili powder, paprika, and cumin until soft,

about 3 minutes. Add kale and cook until soft,

about 2 minutes. Stir in marinara sauce and season

with salt and pepper; turn off the pot and let cool for 5 minutes.

Crack eggs carefully in the pot, evenly spaced. Close and lock the lid. Select low pressure according to manufacturer's instructions; set timer for 1 minute. Once it beeps, release pressure carefully using the quick-release method according to manufacturer's instructions, about 2 minutes. Unlock and remove the lid. Sprinkle with parsley.

Nutrition Facts :

Per Serving: 123 calories; 8.2 g fat; 6.7 g carbohydrates; 6.8 g protein; 164 mg cholesterol; 298 mg sodium.

Recipe Four: Sufganiyot (Dessert)

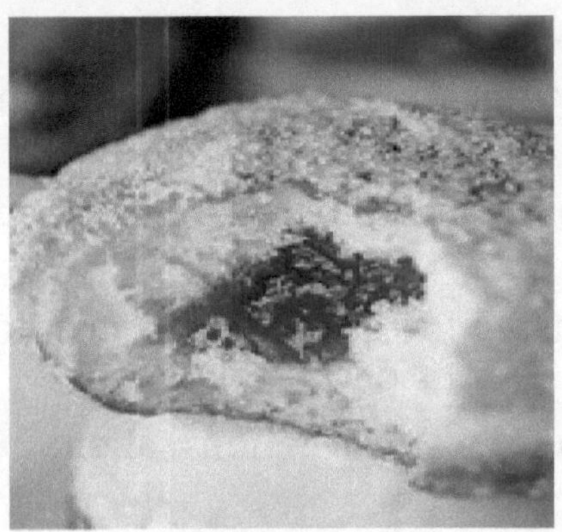

dslot%201

"Doughnuts without holes! This is a traditional Jewish holiday recipe; sufganiyot are commonly served during the Hanukkah season." This traditionally was like a jelly filled doughnut filled with jelly.

Ingredients

4 cups self-rising flour

2 eggs

2 (8 ounce) containers yogurt

Yoplait Black Cherry French Style Yogurt 5 Oz

2 tablespoons white sugar

1 pinch salt

2 tablespoons vanilla sugar

3 quarts vegetable oil for frying

Directions:

Combine flour, eggs, yogurt, sugar, salt and vanilla sugar in a large mixing bowl. Mix well. Set the dough aside for 30 minutes.

Form the dough into balls with a 2-inch diameter.

Heat the vegetable oil to 365 degrees F (190

degrees C) in a large pot or deep fryer over high

heat. It is best to use a basket or slotted spoon for

deep frying the sufganiyot, as the oil will be

extremely hot. Deep fry the dough in the oil. Let

the sufganiyot cool and drain on paper towels.

Recipe Five: Cholent

Kosher Cholent Recipe

Recipe by: Sherrie D.

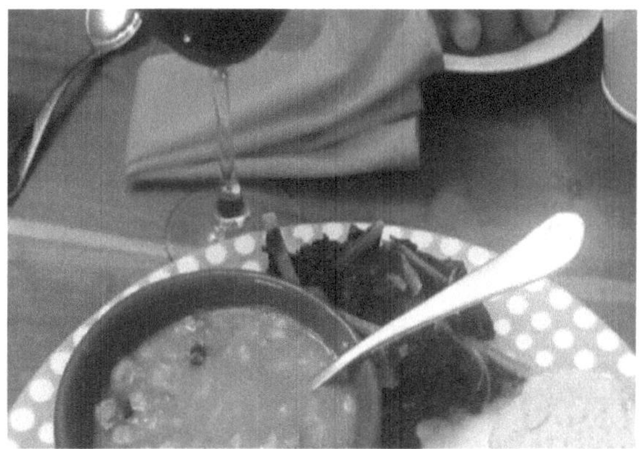

"This is a very filling and hearty stew. It cooks slowly overnight for a minimum of 10 to 15 hours or more on a very low flame." It is all about keeping the Shabbat! Since no electric is the rule of the Shabbat this recipe is started on Friday and done for Shabbat.

Sometimes, it is paired with bread called

Challah Bread.

Ingredients:

3 onions, quartered

4 tablespoons vegetable oil

4 pounds chuck roast, cut into large chunks

1 cup dry kidney beans

1 cup dried pinto beans

1 cup pearl barley

5 large potatoes, peeled and cut into thirds

boiling water to cover

2 (1 ounce) packages dry onion and
mushroom soup mix

2 tablespoons garlic powder

salt and pepper to taste

In a large oven safe pot or roasting pan, saute onions in oil over medium heat.

Add meat, and brown well on all sides.

Mix in beans; stir continuously until the beans start to shrivel. Stir in the barley. Add potatoes, and add just enough boiling water to cover the meat and potatoes. Mix in dry soup mix and garlic. Season with salt and pepper. Bring to a boil, lower heat, and simmer partially covered for 20 minutes on stove top.

Preheat oven to 200 degrees F (95 degrees C).

Cover pot tightly, and place in preheated oven. Allow to cook overnight for at least 10 to 15 hours. Check periodically to make sure you have enough liquid to cover; add small amounts of water if needed. Do not stir; stirring will break up the chunks of potatoes.

Nutrition Facts:

Per Serving: 1067 calories; 49.2 g fat; 98.3 g carbohydrates; 58 g protein; 161 mg cholesterol; 616 mg sodium.

Additional Resources

·   Published Titles:

·   <u>Finding Healing in God's Backyard: Teaching Edition</u>

·   <u>Finding Healing in God's Backyard: Student Edition</u>

·   <u>Depressed Super-Heroes of The Bible</u>

·   <u>Birds of the Bible</u>

·   <u>Essential Oils and Remedies Found in God's Backyard</u>

·   <u>The Little Book of Christmas Plays</u>

·   <u>What Advent Isn't! 6 weeks of Christian Advent   Celebrations</u>

Several of my YouTube videos:

https://youtu.be/mBN9_WcA_fA

How to get paid in DōTERRA.

https://youtu.be/7YCpRLS2jCs

The secret to closing the BEST a show!

https://youtu.be/olVMTM7KY6Q

Alcohol Free Hand Sanitizer

https://youtu.be/x64LA_CQc8I

Get the most FREE with DōTERRA.

https://youtu.be/OvAPDlx2Q34

Do I want both Essential Oil books?

https://youtu.be/_8gSH9md2z8

Why should I be a DōTERRA Advocate?

https://youtu.be/-Qmw0UseQ40

Why I wrote Finding Healing in God's Backyard.

https://youtu.be/_k2joaS9GLY

What Is the Birds of the Bible about?

https://youtu.be/mBN9_WcA_fA

How to get paid with DōTERRA.

https://youtu.be/CiOz3jIiKx8

Dry Chapped skin

https://youtu.be/p9SNjE03k0A

Eating Healthy with essential oils

https://youtu.be/xQ_vFzXXE4w

New book release: Depressed.

https://youtu.be/3hfBaL8abkY Book Trailer

https://youtu.be/JP2EiCRK2Uo Book Trailer

https://youtu.be/yqDmm64D2T8 Book Trailer

https://youtu.be/eXi7LBrhHlM How to save $800 in one year

1. http://10373.createlastingsuccess.com/10373-1534756095

Work at Home ad! Request your free eBook!

2. http://10373.createlastingsuccess.com/10373-149617042012795 0217

Request your free guide on what are essential oils!

3. Book release: Landing Page Ad:

http://10373.createlastingsuccess.com/10373-149426918756535 6536

4. http://rejuvinatemyselfnow.com/10373-817685203

Landing page for book releases

Christian Faith Books Webpages for my books:

http://www.christianfaithpublishing.com/books/?book=findin -healing-in-gods-backyard-student-edition

http://www.christianfaithpublishing.com/books/?book=finding-healing-in-gods-backyard

Press Releases:

Finding Healing in God's Backyard: Student Edition" from Christian Faith Publishing author

Jessica Linhart is a guide to the essential oils featured in the Bible. This guide teaches readers about the healing properties of essential oils and their religious significance while serving as an invaluable resource for Bible study.

http://www.christianfaithpublishing.com/client/301449/301449Linhart-PRrelease.pdf?draft=2017-06-13-05

"Finding Healing in God's Backyard" from Christian Faith Publishing author Jessica Linhart is a comprehensive guide to the properties and use of "God's medicine"- the same essential oils utilized in many passages in Scripture.

http://www.christianfaithpublishing.com/client/301

448/301448Linhart-PRrelease.pdf?draft=2017-06-

13-43

Additional Websites:

www.findinghealinginGodsbackyard.com/store

www.biblical-bookmarks.blog

www.mydoterra.com/craftyfarmer

Bible study one
https://youtu.be/VMDqYRGnpnI

Antointing oils
https://youtu.be/uGV8fBVp1yI

DIY hand sanitizer
https://youtu.be/J_AYIXTqbQI

Mouth wash & Toothpaste

https://youtu.be/9lvCKADZZlc

Make up remover wipes and cleanser

https://youtu.be/xrqv5tDltBs

God's grace anointing oil

https://youtu.be/YLVushicWGY

Elijah

https://youtu.be/by3TsJX_1Eo

Queen Esther

https://youtu.be/GBqmiPRN5Zg

Hyssop

https://youtu.be/C35CJuN0I64

Oil of Joy and Gladness

https://youtu.be/C_tnutfhJ-M

Why should Christians use Essential Oils

https://youtu.be/t6PS0nkGEfc

Universal Prayer Blend

https://youtu.be/Bcb5TynXtHk

Purging fire anointing oil

https://youtu.be/kc4zMI5qHwg

10 beliefs of a CHRISTIANs

https://youtu.be/uLQcSH7xd28

Gruesome events of scripture that you won't hear in church.

https://youtu.be/lP_3OeEP4SE

How to make Jesus's whip

https://youtu.be/k5nCeBYYIeU

Hepatitis A and handwashing

https://youtu.be/TEczHszeJR8

Learn how to live a salty life

https://youtu.be/jdRalkjBF5A

Why do Muslims hate Christians?

https://youtu.be/oRnd33Sv-GQ

Encouragement from a boat

https://youtu.be/ySMQNPQa_w0

Three gruesome deaths in the Bible

https://youtu.be/NYp_oC_cwUg

How to care for a sting naturally?

https://youtu.be/LAagSfUi4pc

What does the locus mean in Bible prophecy?

https://youtu.be/bvFdUnmFQ3k

What is the Bdellium?

https://youtu.be/_GsnXydULO0

What are the best essential oil's for leather?

https://youtu.be/ZwiqyeBp4KI

Learn to pray!

https://youtu.be/OH6-fR4uy9A

What is perfume in Scripture?

https://youtu.be/-V9Zvo-aYzQ

What are essential oils

https://youtu.be/fCnraHaKrV0

Anointing Jesus's feet

https://youtu.be/kl7S7QHOcIo

Myrrh and Spikenard

https://youtu.be/U2sasxQqGXM

Balm of Gilead

https://youtu.be/0nh-ekBZNA0

The Altar Anointing Oil

https://youtu.be/h3mC9XBLMr8